This is a guided journal and wc
Practitioners. Reiki 2 Symbols
instruction in order to access the energies in a reliable way.
From your training, draw and name the three Reiki Level 2
Symbols here for reference.

What areas of your life could use a light switch activation? How would you recognize this "activation"? Draw a Reiki Power Symbol next to each description and repeat "Cho Ku Rei" three times.

What does empowerment mean to you? Practice drawing the Reiki Power Symbol while imagining your empowered self. Whenever you think of your desired outcome, mentally see, say and draw Cho Ku Rei.

Choose your favorite or least favorite room. Draw the Reiki Power Symbol in each corner of the room, upper and lower, while silently chanting "Cho Ku Rei" three times at each corner. How did the energy of the room feel before and after?

With eyes closed, feel your body and follow your breath. Does any area feel tired or weak? Draw an image or insert a photo of yourself below. Place Cho Ku Rei over each area of concern. What do you notice? Use your hands to send the symbol into your body. How do you feel? What did you learn?

Consider situations that drain you. How can Cho Ku Rei represent needed boundaries or support? (Stamped on a closing door? As a drain stopper? Tattooed on a helping hand?) Experiment to learn which ideas work best in each situation.

What are your personal life mottos? Which Reiki 2 Symbol(s) support(s) these mottos? Draw the symbol(s) next to each motto while chanting the symbol name(s).

How will you remind yourself to use Reiki 2 Symbols when you feel tired, anxious or drained? Get creative!

Choose an object to infuse with Reiki. Record your intention (i.e. protection, healing, inspiration, strength, relaxation). Which Reiki 2 Symbol(s) represent your intention? See, say and draw the symbol(s) over your chosen object. Whenever you wear or touch this object, it will convey that quality of Reiki energy.

Make a list of seven things for which you feel grateful. What little (or big) miracles have you experienced? As you practice drawing Cho Ku Rei, fill your heart with gratitude.

In what ways do you feel mentally and emotionally balanced? In which areas could you use more harmony between thoughts and feelings? As you practice drawing the Mental Emotional Balance symbol, mentally repeat "Sei Heki" (say hay kee) three times for each drawing. How do you feel after drawing and saying this symbol?

What does the phrase "God and humanity become one" mean to you? As you practice drawing the Harmony symbol, mentally repeat "Sei Heki" (say hay kee) three times for each symbol.

How do you recognize the Divine moving through your life? Which habits open or slow the flow? When you need Divine inspiration, how can you remind yourself to see, say and draw Sei Heki?

What patterns, addictions or habits would you like to improve? As you practice drawing the Mental Emotional Balance Symbol, repeat "Sei Heki" three times for each symbol. Draw a Sei Heki symbol next to each of the areas you wish to improve. Record your insights.

Stand up and make the Mental Emotional Balance Symbol using wide arm strokes, almost like a dance. Repeat Sei Heki as a mantra, silently or aloud as you embody the symbol. In the space below, ponder any blocks or resistance you may have towards healing. See, say and draw Sei Heki, while intending their release. Record your insights.

In which areas of life do you experience reactivity? What's the difference between reacting, responding, and embracing? How can you use Sei Heki to redirect your energy?

How do your own experiences of reactivity or imbalance fit into the larger collective? As you practice drawing Sei Heki, imagine and intend healing for yourself and our world.

What do "peace," "serenity" and "spirit" mean to you? Place one hand on your heart and one on the top of your head. Mentally see, say and draw Sei Heki. Breathe slowly while you run this symbol through your head and heart. Record any observations below.

Create a collage or drawing that symbolizes peace, serenity and spirit. Physically or mentally draw and repeat Sei Heki above or alongside these images.

Offer Reiki to your feet, either "hands on" or "beaming" Reiki and the Sei Heki Symbol to your feet. How does a "balanced, grounded foundation" look or feel?

Practice drawing the Reiki Distant Healing Symbol. Does it help to count each stroke? Say "Hon She Ze Sho Nen" (HONE-shah-ZAY-show-NEN) as you draw the symbol.

Stand up and practice drawing the Reiki Distant Healing Symbol in wide strokes, moving your hands and arms like a dance. How does it feel to embody Hon Sha Ze Sho Nen?

"The Buddha in me reaches out to the Buddha in you to promote enlightenment and peace." What does this statement mean to you? Practice drawing Hon Sha Ze Sho Nen and record any additional insights.

How do you experience time? When does time fly or drag? Practice drawing, dancing and saying Hon Sha Ze Sho Nen. What does "no past, no present, no future" mean to you?

Where would you love to travel and why? Mentally see, say, draw Hon Sha Ze Sho Nen and imagine being there. The Distant Healing Symbol creates a portal. Watch for synchronicities.

What are your personal ethics around sending Reiki? What does "Highest Good of All" mean, and how might this influence your Reiki practice?

Write down a past or future event. See, say and physically draw the Reiki Distant Healing symbol above and around this event. Pay attention to any memories, emotions or synchronicities you experience. Make a habit of acknowledging and recording results.

Draw the Reiki Distant Healing Symbol and silently chant "Hon Sha Ze Sho Nen" three times. With your left hand, send Reiki to a past trauma or root cause, infusing that event with Reiki. With your right hand, send Reiki to the remedy or desired positive outcome. Record any insights or ideas.

Do you believe everything happens for a reason? Use Sei Heki and Hon Sha Ze Sho Nen together to enhance discernment. What words, images, dreams or coincidences come to mind?

In which state do you experience the strongest flow of Reiki? Which Reiki symbols or techniques help you to "let go and let God"?

What does "no time, no space" mean to you? Think of someone in a different location than you. Repeat their name and "Hon Sha Ze Sho Nen" three times.

Experiment with seeing/saying/drawing Cho Ku Rei before you use the Reiki Distant Healing Symbol. Practice drawing both symbols while mentally chanting their names. Think of a time in the past or future when you could use extra empowerment and send Cho Ku Rei to that time.

In what ways do you embody a need for generational healing? With names, photos, or family tree, use Hon Sha Ze Sho Nen to send Reiki to your ancestors for the highest good of all, including you and future generations.

Create a list of goals or a mini vision board on this page. Embed the Reiki 2 Symbols that address your goals into, under or around your words and images.

What are your fears or phobias? Experiment with each Reiki Level 2 Symbol to bring courage, peace, and/or healing across time and space.

What are your attitudes about giving and receiving? Which Reiki 2 Symbol(s) would help to foster healing and balanced exchange?

How do you feel about money? Invite Universal Life Force Energy to flow through your finances. Which symbol(s) feel most aligned with your prosperity?

Are you happy with your body? Why or why not? Which of the Reiki 2 Symbols supports a healthier experience? How will you practice Reiki to support your physical, mental, emotional and spiritual health?

What and whom would you include in a Reiki Box? Create one in your mind or in physical form, embedding it with resonant symbols and intentions.

In which areas do you already teach by modeling? How could the Reiki 2 Symbols offer empowerment, balance and/or healing in your role as a teacher?

What happens to worry when you express gratitude? What happens to anxiety when you send Reiki to the cause of your anxiety? Experiment and note your trends.

"The Divine in me reaches out to the Divine in you to create enlightenment and peace." What does this statement tell you about Distant Healing?

This journal has ended, but the journey continues. You can find more information on Reiki, healing and intuition at http://asklaurabruno.com . Reiki blessings to you and yours!

Made in the USA
Middletown, DE
08 July 2019